My Long Road to Freedom

by

Jenny Chapman

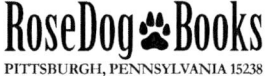

PITTSBURGH, PENNSYLVANIA 15238

The contents of this work including, but not limited to, the accuracy of events, people, and places depicted; opinions expressed; permission to use previously published materials included; and any advice given or actions advocated are solely the responsibility of the author, who assumes all liability for said work and indemnifies the publisher against any claims stemming from publication of the work.

All Rights Reserved
Copyright © 2017 by Jenny Chapman

No part of this book may be reproduced or transmitted, downloaded, distributed, reverse engineered, or stored in or introduced into any information storage and retrieval system, in any form or by any means, including photocopying and recording, whether electronic or mechanical, now known or hereinafter invented without permission in writing from the publisher.

RoseDog Books
585 Alpha Drive
Suite 103
Pittsburgh, PA 15238
Visit our website at *www.rosedogbookstore.com*

ISBN: 978-1-4809-7030-4
eISBN: 978-1-4809-7007-6

My Long Road to Freedom

Early Memories

I was born in 1941, in November. At the age of three my memory served me very well.

I would often lie on the floor and scream by the hour, and also scream in front of company. I remember on one occasion being offered sweets, but I still screamed. I did stop before my mother and I left for home, and we came home through the forest. My mother sat down on a log with me on her lap. Cuddling me she cried bitterly, "Why do you scream so much"?

Another time in company I tried to hide by curling up in the chair behind my mother. One lady said, "She needs a brother". This too I remember to this day.

It was at this age that I awoke one night to find my father under my bedclothes seeking sexual gratification. I was mortified, and knew this to be naughty. I was frozen to the bed, too frightened to breathe.

As an adult I read about a girl who had an identical experience, and cried out to her father "Go away you dirty beast!" However in my situation I was far too scared. I was speechless. Had I said this, my father's violent temper would erupt over something quite different. He would beat my mother, and on one occasion threw hot ashes on the kitchen floor. I was scared of him, and I had no respect for him. I thought he had been very naughty to get under my bedclothes.

I had my first visit to an optician at the age of three. I had a squint in both eyes. I was filled with horror. No one explained anything to me. So when a large frame designed to hold different lenses was placed on my nose, I thought that these were my new glasses. However, I wore my real glasses on the end of my nose for quite some time. It was glasses that led me to being called "four eyes". Few children wore glasses at my age.

I was born during World War Two. The air raid siren, was terrifying. It had a sound that just droned on and on calling everyone to dive for cover. I would hate that sound even now, if it was brought to life.

I remember being bundled into the tiny cupboard under the stairs. We had to arrange ourselves around various household items such as the carpet sweeper, and other commodities. It was dark, very cramped, and rather spidery.

Later we upped our game and had an indestructible Morrison shelter. This was placed in the lounge. It became our den for the three of us, when the air raid was sounded. Father and Mother slept side by side with me by their heads. I really thought that it was quite cosy, and so much nicer than that horrid cupboard under the stairs.

Then, of course, there were the blackout curtains covering every window in the house. If the enemy detected a chink of light, then he would reward us with one of his bombs.

My grandparents lived in Ramsgate, Kent. They had what was known as a dugout, situated in their garden. This was very damp, because it was under ground. It smelt very musty, and was full of spiders, and plenty of other creepy crawlies. I remember the air raid siren sounding in the night. I was scared so I usually sought safety under the bedclothes. Then I would be carried to the dugout. We were joined by the neighbours. We were quite happy, sitting by candlelight. It was a bit scary, and very creepy. I remember on one occasion, the all clear was sounded, and my mother carrying me up into the daylight, and pointed to a glorious sunrise. It was like a beacon of hope.

One morning my mother showed me the sea for the first time. I was three. I exclaimed that it was just a big bath. I was also taken down onto the sand for the first time. It was full of tiny insects crawling and flying all over the sand. This made such an impact on me, that when it came to breakfast the next morning, I refused to eat my cereal because I thought the strands were the insects that I had seen on the sand. However, discipline was such that I sat there until I had eaten the cereal, even though I was screaming. Then I refused strawberries, because I thought the pips were insects. These made me scream.

When I was three my brother John was born. I am very fond of him, and we were always good pals as children. We played and we went out together. Later, we went to the swimming pool on our bikes. We had an ice lolly on the way home, and sat in the local graveyard to enjoy. We chose a different grave stone each time. Somehow we found this very amusing. On one occasion we thought a grave looked too small, so we tested it for size by lying on it.

My father had made up his mind that he was going to have another girl and was, apparently quite annoyed when my brother was born. For obvious reasons he wanted a girl. Not to be loved in the right sense, but to be used as I was. He would take quite bizarre opportunities to uncover my shame. Looking back, I do wonder why my mother did not become aware of his behaviour in this matter. She let me down in this way.

At some point, I did let tell my grandmother, on my Mother's, side about my father, and what he did to me. I do not know to this day what 1 told her. I rather think that I possibly blurted it out. My grandmother was a lovely quiet person. She would listen, but not say much. You could say anything to her. She had such a sympathetic ear. Both my grandparents tackled my mother over this issue. My mother just said that my father would not do such things. So she let me down again.

My father, and also his father, both had bipolar affective disorder, and at a very young age, my father was aware that I also had this disorder. He did point this out to my mother. However, this disorder did not excuse him for being the paedophile that he so obviously proved to be.

World War Two ended, but the legacy it left continued for many years. The noise from planes and the trains always sent me running indoors for a sense of safety. Steam trains passed at the end of our garden, they were very noisy. There were sidings at the end of our garden. At night the trains would shunt backwards and forwards, making a dreadful noise. They rattled as they crashed into each other. Sometimes a torch would light up my bedroom. I would be so scared that I would call out to my parents for reassurance. For years, I was scared to make a trip to the toilet in case there was someone outside my bedroom. Perhaps someone would creep in from the trains.

One day my mother and I were on the station platform when a train full of trucks passed by. I asked my mother what they were called. I thought she said that they were Gods train. I was puzzled for sometime as to why God should have such an awful train. I was only three.

I remember the ration books. The war caused a shortage of food. A coupon was exchanged for a food product, and even sweets were rationed.

We made many clothes. Knitting wool was scarce, and we would often come by a bundle of wool. This had to be unravelled and picked, until it could be made into a ball of wool. Often jumpers would be unpicked so as to make the correct quantity for whatever purpose.

I had striped jumpers. 1 had a striped bathing costume, which when wet fell to my knees in a soggy mass. Even my vests and socks were hand knitted.

When it came to Christmas and birthdays, many presents were made by hand. Coat hangers were covered in pieces of material. Table cloths were embroidered, as were other items. Garments were knitted. Jam was made. Second hand books were bought for presents, but they were sterilized in the oven first to rid them of disease.

One Christmas my grandfather made me a wonderful dolls house, along with all the furniture. My grandmother made the little dolls.

Presents in those days were truly valued and appreciated. They were often planned well before Christmas, and involved much time and thought. Some presents that had been purchased were often very basic and even crude. Money was short, but we were always thankful with what we had been given.

Everyone was encouraged to grow their own vegetables, to help overcome the food shortage. This not only provided food for us but also healthy exercise.

Very few people had a car. We just walked. My mother often took me out for walks. On one occasion, my mother wheeled my pram, but 1 just refused to use it, as I was happy to walk. In later years I worked out that I had in fact walked about six miles.

In those days men and women nearly always wore hats when out and about. Women mostly wore dresses or skirts, along with stockings, and shoes made from leather, as did the men.

Each home had a pantry in the kitchen to store food. Flies invariably found their way in, and if food was not covered and the flies had laid eggs, these were picked off later.

The weekly washing was done in a huge copper boiler. This took up a lot of space in the kitchen. After the wash, the water was squeezed out of the washing by a large mangle. It was operated by a handle which turned two big rollers that, as they turned, took the washing through, squeezing out the water. When the mangle was packed away it then became our kitchen table. There was, of course, very little leg room. If it was a dry day, the washing was hung in the garden on a cotton line. Sometimes this line would snap, sending the washing onto the ground. Then the washing often had to be done again, if necessary. On wet days the washing would be draped over wooden rails hanging from the kitchen ceiling making the whole kitchen feel very damp.

Of course we had no central heating. In fact we had never even heard of it. We had a coal fire burning in the evening in the lounge, which we sat round to keep warm. We also had a coke boiler in the kitchen, which I think was to heat the water. On a bitterly cold morning we would all dress in the kitchen by the boiler and the oven, which was lit for extra warmth.

Bananas were not seen until after the war, and even then they were in very short supply. So although I was only allowed half a banana it was still a huge treat.

I must not forget the lamp lighter, with his ladder. He came down our road every evening to light our street lights.

I was three when my mother showed me a very untidy cupboard. As I looked into it, I did exclaim that it was just a muddle. This was the birth of a very tidy mind that continues to this day.

I remember with much affection my dear aunty Ethel. She lived with us for a time during the war. She was a skilled dressmaker, which she did by profession, and also made many clothes for me. However, she did have an artificial leg. Owing to T.B one leg was amputated. She would walk a great distance to get to church, although she was very wary of wet leaves. She was tiny, a little round, and very quiet and very cuddly. I always called her arty.

I Start School

I was very proud to be starting school, and I told my parents to call me school girl, but that fell on deaf ears.

Weeks before starting school, I contracted whooping cough, so I did not attend on the first day. Instead I had weeks of coughing and sickness.

My mother took me to school. I do not know what her feelings were, but I skipped down the stairs, and turned to wave goodbye. I was very happy. My father was very proud. So my brother and I were sent to private schools I did not attend a good school. On reflection, the headmistress did everything to cut corners to save money. The teachers were elderly, and possibly not paid a good wage.

My mother wanted us to attend the local council school. Looking back, this would have been a better option, but my mother had to give way to my father. She was a very shy timid person, but latterly became extremely stubborn.

I was rather withdrawn at school. I felt detached. I would cry if the teacher read a sad story.

Once a week we cut pictures from a magazine. I so enjoyed this, and I had good control with the scissors. I felt very proud one lesson to be given a large picture of the Queen. Perhaps this was the birth of my love of art and craft.

I loved singing lessons. One lesson the teacher had a coughing fit. She left the room to get a glass of water, and on her return was greeted with a chorus, "We thought you were going to die".

In winter the classroom was heated by a lovely coal fire. The small bottles of milk that we had each day had to be placed in front of the fire on a bitterly cold day. On these days we kept our coats on. Of course if you sat near the fire the warmer you became. However, a brisk run around the playground soon warmed us. I put this tactic into action when I was teaching, even if at the side of the desks in the form of physical jerks.

At Christmas we all sat round the fire. The teacher made each of us a little gift, which she placed in a stocking. I had a blue comb in a felt case.

One morning, in my next year, I asked to go to the toilet. I looked through a glass door, and saw a girl being taught the violin. I sat entranced as I listened and just wished that was me. I memorised the time and day of the lesson, and each week I made a point of asking to go to the toilet. I would listen for as long as I dared. I never dreamed then that many years later that I would be playing a violin.

At the age of eight I began to teach myself to play our piano. My mother had taught me one or two little ditties, and this had spurred me on. I had my first piano book, and I taught myself the notes, and little pieces. Possibly badly, I do not know.

Then we had those very thick fogs. They were called pea soups. At times you could not see your hand in front of you.

So much took place when I was about eight. I had my tonsils removed, which gave me such a sore throat for a week.

I had my first bike. I sailed out of the shop and up the pavement. My parents were rather surprised, but I had already learnt to ride my friends little bike.

My brother started school, and my parents decided that as my numerical skills were so poor, I might do better if I attended the same school. It was a private school mainly for boys. There was just one other girl in my class. The boys had accepted her, but they never accepted me. As I took my seat on that first morning, I was frightened and bewildered. There was a chorus from some of the boys. "Look behind you!" All eyes were on me, full of hostility that remained with me until I left the school.

I was given the nickname of Smelly. Every morning when I entered the classroom the boys threw my possessions out of the classroom window. I was frequently hit so hard that I was winded. If I retaliated in any way, it would be reported to the teachers and I would get into trouble. I just welled up and couldn't speak up to defend myself.

One morning, at the age of eight, I told my mother that I had a tummy ache. That meant a day off school. I was taken to the doctor, who diagnosed appendicitis. I had a whole week off school to rest before going into hospital to have them removed. Unfortunately, this episode led me to realize that illness got me out of school, and also gained me the attention I craved.

I was excited to be taken to hospital by ambulance, and my mother certainly encouraged this. Perhaps this was unwise.

The day of the surgery was very traumatic. I remembered the day I had my tonsils removed. Now I had to face it again. I retched over the medicine, and knocked the gas mask off my face. I awoke from the surgery stiff and sore. I was lonely in a ward of four old ladies. Well, old to me.

Visitors brought me sweets and chocolate, but being self conscious I ate under the bedclothes. I often had a good cry there as well.

Every day a nurse came round to each patient, and asked us if we had opened our bowels. I had no idea what she was talking about. So I said yes one day, and no the next. Even so, I was given a laxative, which was very unpleasant.

Many years later, I was told that the surgeon had found nothing wrong with my appendix, but not knowing this I still complained of stomach ache. So at the age of eight I saw a psychiatrist. He asked me if I liked school, and I said that I hated it. He advised my mother to send me to a girl's school, and in fact I was able to return to my first school.

I had learnt to be a tomboy. On my first morning I yelled the first words of the Lord's Prayer in assembly. Another morning two staff were talking on the stairs, blocking my access, so I slid down the banisters. I was reprimanded for this.

At the age of eight I always tried to do my best in everything. I always had to win. My brother had quite a different approach to life. Because of this he had so much encouragement in everything, and I very little. I think my parents assumed that as I mastered things, I did not need this.

There was one thing in my life that I did treasure. That was my bedroom. It was mine. I could escape there and be alone.

At the age of eight, my world was shattered. My mother told me that another baby was on the way.

As a child, I worried over many things. All of which I kept to myself, and were possibly quite unfounded.

When my grandparents came to stay with us, they slept in my bedroom. I worried that when they were very old, that they would have to live with us and have my room.

Sometimes, my brother had to sleep with me in my room. I resented this as he sucked his fingers very noisily. So I threw books at him, in revenge.

Another baby would mean that I would lose my room. On reflection, my father wanted another girl.

As time went on, my mother became bed bound. The neighbour next door to us came each day to help prepare meals.

My brother and I were sent to our grandparents in Ramsgate. We were extremely naughty, and even reduced my grandmother to tears .My mother had gone into hospital and later joined us in Ramsgate. There was no explanation, and nothing was said to me. However, I knew within me, that now there would be no baby.

I learnt in later years that my mother had a mole. This meant no more babies. If my father felt let down, he overcame this in a very evil way.

One day when I was about eight, we met up with another family, and had a picnic in the local woods. I was given a small bowl, and went to pick blackberries. I was enjoying this, when a man appeared out of the bush and asked me what I was doing. He told me that he knew where there were some very big blackberries. I was thrilled to hear this, and happily trotted along with him. I chatted as I went, but he never spoke to me. We came to a bush, and he pushed me into it. By now I was scared. He partly undressed me, and played about with me in a disgusting manner. As he started to take my cardigan off, I pulled my arms out and fled, screaming, out of the bush. I soon got back to my mother, and told her the whole story. She did not really comfort me, but rather casually said that there wasn't much point in telling the police as the man would have run off by now. So we just went home.

This episode has always remained with me. Even now, I will not walk alone in woods, or lonely places. I still tend to look behind me when few people are about.

One year when we were on holiday with my grandparents, my mother had to take me to the doctor. It so happened that I saw the same doctor that she had seen when she was living with her parents. My mother had become very large by the time I was eight. The doctor exclaimed how big she was now, then looked at me and said, "In twenty years time you will be as big as your mother." That stuck, and the seed was sown for anorexia nervosa which took over my life when I was in my twenties.

I would argue that if I did not eat too much then I would not get fat. The family would hit back that the doctor said I would, and after all he knew. I started to look at myself and compare my body to my friends. If someone was thinner than me, then I was envious. So at that age I wanted to be slim.

It was at college at the age of twenty that I was weighed and told that I should try and lose a few pounds. It was that silly woman that triggered the anorexia that had laid dormant all those years.

In general, life was very different in those days. I always cycled to school. Home for dinner, then back for afternoon school. People generally had their main meals midday.

Shopping was totally different. We did not have cars. So we walked to the nearest shops. There was a greengrocer, a grocers shop, a bakers shop, a hardware shop, and quite often a wool shop. Food was not covered, as it is today. One day when we were at a market the hot cross buns were piled high on a stall. They had no covering. We survived.

Further Struggles

As I became older, I was aware of the strict religion, or sect, that was part of my life. This was instigated by a man known as J.N. Darby. It was called the Plymouth Brethren. They even had their own Bible. I was bitter and resentful of the shame and anguish that this put me through, throughout most of my life.

We did not talk about going to church, but rather, to the meeting. There was some trouble in the early years with this religion, but as time went on it grew steadily worse. It took the form of an ever increasing number of very strict rules. These made me feel like a social outcast. I had nothing in common with my classmates at school. At home we were not allowed to have a radio, a television or even a record player. I couldn't go to the cinema. I was not allowed to wear trousers. I had to have long hair, which was not fashionable at the time. When I went out my head had to be covered with a hat and later in life with a headscarf. In fact, we were not to be in any way conformed to the world. To me this was a horrendous situation.

Sometimes when I was out walking alone, I would kick stones, asking myself why I had been born to parents belonging to the Plymouth Brethren. There were, to my mind, plenty of sensible religions abounding that I could see nothing wrong with.

I dreaded Sunday. On Saturday I felt physically ill, because the next day was Sunday. Saturday was bath night, and my hair was washed. Because it was so long it was a horrid experience, and it was for many years to come.

Sunday arrived with the usual palaver. Clean underwear, clean socks, my best dress, best coat, best hat, and gloves. Everyone in this meeting had to look better than anyone else. It was a stiff competition.

So thus, I was walked through the streets. I felt stupid, and fearful that I might see a classmate from school. In summer I had to wear a frightful straw hat, with artificial flowers that my mother had sewn on. If my brother could wear his school cap, then why could I not wear my school beret?

Very strict rules were imposed on me throughout Sunday. I was only allowed to play hymns on the piano. I could not knit, or sew, or read novels. Sunday had to be holy. I was constantly reminded to take care of my best clothes, and also that it was Sunday. As if I could forget. On Sunday I felt as though I had been screwed down in my coffin. The relief when that day was over. I could fly like a bird, up and away from it. That is until next Saturday.

I was not allowed to play, or go into the homes of anyone who did not belong to our religion. I might have been contaminated, I don't know why else.

Eventually, as time went on, and I was even older, I was made to endure three meetings every Sunday, and three meetings in the week, in the evening. I dreaded all these meetings, because of their length, and therefore the extreme boredom that they incurred on me. The clocks seemed at a standstill.

Sunday, which we had to call Lord's Day, began with communion, or, in other words the breaking of bread, to us. One had to qualify to take part in this event, and had to go through a lengthy questionnaire from someone considered more holy than anyone else in the gathering. Anyone in disgrace was excluded from this activity and therefore had to sit at the back of the room in future. They were not even spoken to, but treated as outcasts. This was not right. No one was perfect, and many resorted to adultery, as a way of breaking down the austerity in the regime.

This included my father. He was also excluded, and he did not take to it quietly. To my utter shame, he would at times storm into the room in a temper and shout obscenities. My mother would leave the room to usher him out, leaving me alone and rigid with shame.

Once a month on a Saturday evening, there was a care meeting. This was supposed to deal with the business affairs. The leader of this religion was a relatively wealthy man usually living, as far as I can remember, in America. So every care meeting, and all over the world, the Plymouth Brethren sent their leader a sum of money. On reflection, I can think of many individuals and families who were struggling financially, or even on the breadline, who were given no help at all financially. How wrong this was.

I soon learnt that any illness meant that I could stay home on Sunday. This made me happy. I was allowed to draw and paint pictures and I enjoyed that. In fact, one Sunday when I was home from college, l started a painting depicting a still life picture. This was eventually shown to the Queen Mother and also helped me gain distinction in art in my finals.

I loved my grandmother, and we seemed like minded. She often said she wished she could take her knitting to these meetings, and it did not take much to make us both giggle.

I was also ashamed of my home. I knew I was different and therefore assumed that my home must also be different to those, say, of my classmates at school. Later in life when I was doing my 'O' levels, a teacher at school offered to give me extra coaching in my home. Shame drove me to decline this kind offer.

I was ashamed of my mother's appearance. Rightly so, I think. In no way did she match up to the other mothers at my private school. This was so apparent on sport days, for example. She was so fat. Her long hair was bound in an untidy bun which hung down her neck. This was topped with a cheap felt hat.

My father had, by now, started bringing young girls home for tea on a Saturday. He had enrolled at a nearby home for children to be an uncle to the girls. This was an evil and wicked thing to do on his part. Many years later I discovered that he took these girls upstairs, undressed them, and took disgusting pornographic photos. He learnt how to develop his own photos, and hid them away. These were discovered many years later after his death. The faces of these girls portrayed the terror that they felt. These girls may well be alive today, and I wonder how they may be feeling.

I was also bathed by my father, until I became of an age to call a halt to this activity.

I had an increased sense of insecurity for many years. I was always so scared if my mother was unwell. I was so afraid that my mother might die and leave me to the mercies of my father. This fear lived with me well into my adult years. I knew that I could not live with my father, and fortunately it did not happen.

At times my father threatened to kill himself. Not that I would have really minded. He would stick his head in the gas oven, but took his head out on the occasion that my grandmother said that it was a pity to waste the gas. Likewise, when he threatened to jump of a bridge, grandmother simply said that it would be a pity to spoil such a nice suit.

I did have a brighter side to my life. At the age of eleven I began piano lessons. I had taught myself as far as the first grade. I liked my teacher, and he taught me well. I loved practicing each day, and I passed my first exams with good marks.

I was soon to start swimming lessons at school. I bought myself a book about swimming, and I hung over the music stool and went through the motions of the breaststroke. 1 soon got the hang of things, and believed that the water would support me. On my first lesson with the school, I entered the water, and I swam. The teacher was very impressed and asked me who had taught me. By the expression on her face, and her reaction, I don't think she believed my answer. You couldn't really blame her.

I very quickly made progress with my swimming. I loved it. My parents would take my brother and me to the nearby open air pool. There the manager taught me all the other strokes, and also taught me how to dive. In my first school swimming sports day I was runner up in the championships. When studying P.E. at college I passed many swimming awards, and took swimming to advanced level in my final year at college. Today I still aim to swim as often as I can at the local pool.

I collected stamps, and took this quite seriously. I saved my pocket money, and took frequent trips to the nearest stamp shop. I would consult the reference books in order to complete sets, or buy more unusual stamps of different countries.

My mother began to nurture a love of nature in me, and this soon took hold. I had a corner of our large garden that was mine. I was given a variety of small flowers. Pansies, with their smiley faces, were my favorite. I neatly planted them all, and kept my little garden weed free and very neat. Just as 1 keep my garden today, and of course now it is all mine.

Eventually, I had my own little vegetable patch. I grew mostly salad plants, and it was always a proud moment when the family tucked into my own products at meal time.

I was taught how to press flowers. Delicately opening out the little leaves and petals, and laying them out between pages in thick books. After about three weeks, I could carefully open the pages to see my flowers or leaves pressed in a way that they would never fade, but last forever. I found this truly remarkable. I then quickly began to learn the names of plants, and this was a life time achievement.

One year at school, in my class, we had a nature competition. My mother helped me make a nature book, very neatly, with pressed plants and flowers. All labeled, with drawings and paintings, and descriptions of their origin. I won that prize, and received a book on flowers that I have to this day.

At the age of eight I had my first camera, a box brownie. Now obsolete, but I was proud of it then. I still have some of those photos even now. I still enjoy the thrill of creating pictures with my camera. It is a form of art in itself.

My dollies were often treated to lavish little parties. I had a dolls china tea set. There was pretend tea and some food that my mother had given me. Of course, I had to eat and drink everything for them, on their behalf.

I used to play at hospital with my dollies. I tucked them all in bed, and treated their wounds. On one occasion, I decided that they needed medicine, because I had that when I was ill. My mother wisely kept this in the top cupboard in the kitchen. It so happened that my parents were in the garden. Undaunted, I managed to place a chair on the draining board, and climbed high enough to reach the medicine. I chose some cough medicine, because I knew it tasted very nice. I gave each doll a very generous dose of medicine, and I had a lot of dolls. I put it to their mouths, and then 1 was very happy to drink it for them. The next morning, my mother had to send for the doctor because she could not rouse me.

My first pet was a little mouse, called Minnie. She was kept in a little cage in the hearth by the fire. One day she was temporarily placed in the garden, in her cage, but long enough for her to find a mate. I placed some cotton wool in her cage, and I was enthralled at the nest she made herself. One day my brother came into the kitchen and announced that Minnie had had a lot of little slugs. What happened to these babies I do not know. They disappeared. A hamster was next. It was not very amusing, apart from climbing up curtains and then falling, with a thud, onto the floor. My brother and I had a rabbit each and we argued for long time over their names. We occasionally brought them indoors, but of course they were not toilet trained, so we had to clean round afterwards. Like many children, we lost interest in them, and it was left to my father to look after them. I now look back with remorse that I didn't care for them as 1 should. My love for creatures is boundless, and they deserve the best. They have a right to their lives. Many times I have picked a worm from the pavement and placed into a garden. I do not stamp on snails, for example, they find pastures new over the fence.

We did not have a car, so we would go on outings, taking a picnic with us. Sometimes we took public transport. There were steam trains, and even trams. On one occasion we walked along railway lines to get to our destination. It seemed in those days that there were no boundaries. We would go fruit picking, and what we didn't eat went in a basket or jam jar. When home, the fruit would be preserved so it could be used in the winter when food was in short supply. Wine was also made from almost anything it seemed. Some even made their beer. It was all a very slow process, and had to be extremely accurate, otherwise it went off and stank.

On fine days, especially on bank holidays, we would put up a tent in the garden. This was always a thrill, because we had a camp fire and cooked sausages. These tasted so much nicer over a smoky fire, than any cooked indoors. I don't think my parents were like minded, but never said so.

One extremely wet bank holiday, we placed our dining table in the front window, and we played snap at every car that went passed the house. We would have to think of something very different today.

I was encouraged to help out with household chores. Every spring, we had what was called spring cleaning. Every room was emptied of furniture. The carpet was taken up. Nobody really had fitted carpets. The carpet was then hung over the washing line and the dust beaten out. Every part of the room and every piece of furniture was scrubbed and polished until it sparkled.

In the garden I learnt how to do some of the tougher jobs. I learnt how to mix concrete and lay paths. We could not afford to have jobs done for us, and this stood me in good stead.

Women did not go out to work. They were housewives, looking after the home and family, and usually the garden as well. Each day of the week had routine. Monday was wash day. Anyone washing late in the week was considered to be slovenly, or even dirty. It was on Monday that the beds were changed. It was lovely that night to get into crisp clean sheets. On Tuesday the ironing was usually done. When I look back at all that had to be ironed, compared to today, there were all the sheets, handkerchiefs, shirts, blouses and even dresses. The house work was fitted in as and when. My mother did all the cooking on Saturday morning, and in the afternoon we did gardening, as far as I remember, the weather did not stop us.

Horse drawn carts often delivered our goods, such as the milk. Any keen gardener would rush out with a paper bag to collect horse droppings, all warm and steaming, to be placed round a precious plant.

Every evening my father brought home the evening paper. I looked forward to this. If one murder had taken place, it was the one and only, and it was the headline.

How different things are today. How far have we really progressed?

Life Goes On

Christmas at home was a thrilling time, and I became excited many weeks beforehand. We made most of our decorations. We would paint a large spray of twigs with white paint, and then hang on our decorations. That was our Christmas tree. We made paper chains with strips of coloured paper and homemade flour paste, which we applied with a brush. It was slow and rather messy but it did give a sense of achievement. We had some rather crude fairy lights shaped like Chinese lanterns, which had been handed down through the generations.

My brother and I went by train to the nearest Woolworths, where we bought our presents for everyone, with our pocket money. We bought little bottles of lavender water, bath salts and similar little gifts. We often got home just as it was getting dark.

We had plenty of carol singers at this time. They were often accompanied by a musical instrument, such as a recorder or even a violin. It was always so festive, and we always looked forward to them at Christmas time.

Our small house was filled with our relatives. Sleeping arrangements were rarely comfortable, but no one minded. I hung my empty stocking by my bed on Christmas Eve, and was too excited to sleep. When I awoke, there was a full, lumpy stocking which I unloaded with my parents and my brother. There were sweets, small toys and little novelties.

Breakfast always consisted of ham, tongue and sausage rolls. Because of our religion, I had to endure a Bible study followed by lengthy prayers. While on our knees, my brother and I made faces each other and tried to stifle our giggles. We thought it a waste of valuable time.

Grandpa dressed as Father Christmas. My brother and I were dressed as pixies or elves. We handed out the presents as they were pulled out of the sack.

Then the anticlimax, as the adults had to go to a religious meeting. They were back for Christmas dinner, which was a lavish affair, with a table full of food and drink. One year a plan was hatched to make me drunk with cider. My head swam and my face became fiery red, and when my mother asked me if I was feeling alright, I lied and said that I was fine. In fact I was worried because I didn't know what was wrong with me.

The rest of the day was spent eating, playing games and charades. We had homemade sweets such as fudge and coconut ice. Many different cakes were made, to suit every ones taste, and of course the Christmas cake. There were plenty of jellies and trifles.

Boxing Day was still fun, but rather an anticlimax. It still is for me today.

In winter, every Saturday evening, we sat round the coal fire at our little tin table. We toasted crumpets over the coal fire and put butter and cheese on them. We always had a big packet of sweets for the evening. Then we spent the time playing different games, such as card games and board games. Needless to say, my sole purpose was to win, rather than just enjoy the games.

In those days, if a doctor was to call this was a big event. The house was tidied and cleaned. He was ushered in almost reverently. If I was ill in bed my mother lit a coal fire in my bedroom as the best way to heat the room. Often, the doctor would warm his hands. The whole road seemed to know if the doctor had called. Sometimes he came on foot, or he came by bicycle. After time, our doctor had his first car.

The doctor was responsible for family health. He would come at night if necessary, usually with his pyjamas under a pair of trousers. One afternoon 1 cut my hand quite badly with a knife, so my father took me to the doctor's home. He knocked on his front door, and I was given the necessary treatment. His surgery was situated within his home. He always made his own prescriptions and placed them on the shelf in the waiting room, for the patients to walk in and collect.

Our local hospital was in fact a cottage hospital. It was small, but well equipped, and dealt with the needs of the local people. There was a matron in a neat uniform in charge, and a kitchen with a cook responsible for the hospital food.

The National Health Service was introduced, as far as I can remember, about the time I was born. Before this medical services had to be paid for. Rather than my granny paying to have her dentures adjusted, she did this with her nail file. My grandpa, who was a carpenter, happened to slice the top of his thumb off one day. Apparently, he picked up the piece of thumb placed it back in position, and bound the thumb with some wood shaving. Unfortunately, he did place the piece the wrong way round, but it healed. As a child, my mother coped with most of my childhood aches and pains, cuts and bruises, just as I try to today.

In my early years, I was encouraged to take on craft work. I learnt basket weaving and modelling. I tried making pictures from different materials. My mother was good at art and craft. She loved painting and craft work and certainly encouraged me to follow that path. I did, and I still enjoy it today.

At the age of eleven every pupil sat the eleven plus examination. This determined whether you went to a grammar school or a secondary modern school. Most of my friends had coaching to pass this examination. I had none. My parents took the attitude that if I failed I would remain at my private school, and they showed no concern as to whether I passed or not. I did fail, and my confidence plunged even further. Of course, I wanted to pass, that was only natural.

I had extra coaching for arithmetic, as I found this so difficult. At times I thought the subject was stupid. Why talk in terms of x or y? Or even as to the amount of liquid in a tub measuring a given size?

My love of sport was paramount, as was my love of music. I gained a place in the netball and hockey teams. I also received my school colours for both, as well as swimming.

I played defence in hockey, and goal shooter in netball. We had matches against other schools, of which I was always proud to be part.

I was not very good at tennis. I played as though my racquet had no strings. I was not able to hit the ball. However, our school had Christine Truman, who became a Wimbledon finalist. She won other championships throughout the world, and also commentated at Wimbledon for many years. She was very tall, and fond of Mars bars. She was quiet and would stand outside the classroom door until the teacher arrived. Her sister, Nell, also attended the school, and I think I am right in saying that they both won the junior championships at Wimbledon. I often met Christine at the Keep Fit group I attended each week. She did say on one occasion that she found it boring, and I certainly did. We tried to do fancy dance steps as though we had climbing boots on our feet, and one session she spent time pulling a long thread on her tights, quite absorbed in unravelling them. It was quite an honour to have her with us. I did meet her when out shopping and we always spoke.

I had a netball post in my garden, and I spent many daylight hours perfecting my shooting skills. I took my netball to school each day, and before school started I went onto the netball court for even more practice. As in everything I worked for perfection rather than sheer pleasure.

I took school sports days very seriously. In fact I dreaded them. I was so afraid that I might get in the wrong team or race, for example.

I have often thought that my mother could have explained to me that it was not the winning that mattered, but the taking part. Also that it was meant to be fun, just a game. I had very little encouragement or praise as a child, unlike my brother .My parents thought that as I achieved things anyway, I didn't need this pat on the back. All children need praise. I, therefore, brought attention to myself in whatever way I could.

As a family we were always short of money. This was down to the private school fees. My mother spent many afternoons at her sewing machine making clothes. She made all my frocks, or dresses, and even coats. To me they looked home made, and again, made me feel different to others. Worse still, my mother bought second - hand clothes from friends for me to wear. I found this very humiliating. However, it was a huge thrill to go into a shoe shop and buy a brand new pair of shoes. In those days we could place our feet in an x ray machine and wriggle our toes in the shoes, for size. It was great to see the bones in my feet.

Snow brought a real thrill to my brother and me. We even wished we lived in Scotland, so that we would have even more. As soon as there was enough of the stuff we took our toboggan to the slopes, and spent hours going up and down. The drag up the hill was more than worth it for the big rush down, to see how far we could reach down the track. There was just one big drawback. Because of my religion, I had to wear a stupid skirt and something on my head. I wore a woolly hat. There were often some from my religion, with their toboggans at the track. I had very little to do with them because their dress was even more ridiculous than mine. Also, I did not wish to be seen with them in case someone from my school happened to be around. They stood out from the crowd that 1 wanted to be part of, as I did in everything else throughout most of my life.

It was so hard at school. I was alone in my private school and this made me miserable, and mixed up. I also felt stupid. All the other school children in my religious gathering went to council schools where they had each other. They all had friends to play with and talk to.

There were various activities arranged amongst those in this religion but as I could not accept the religion, I could not accept those that were part of it.

At school, 1 had to find a way of gaining some recognition. I worked and revised hard in my school work .If I came top, or nearly so, this gave me a sense of pride. 1 had won.

If I devised mischief at school, I stood out from the crowd. I can recall some events. One needlework lesson, I tied a cotton reel on a long enough thread to enable me to swing it so that it tapped on the Headmistress's window below. Our needlework lessons took place in the library, and I was in trouble one lesson, for finding and distributing under the tables some pictures of nudes that 1 had found in some books.

On another occasion, I made a small catapult from some wire and an elastic band. I used it to ping notes around the classroom to other girls. One lesson I misfired, and my note lodged in our teacher's hair. In fact, right in a curl. I was horrified, and this set the girls off giggling, which made the situation even worse. I have no idea what I may have written in the note, or even when it was discovered.

I even went to the effort, along with the girl sitting next to me, of learning some deaf and dumb. We could communicate this way, but not be accused of talking as such.

I think my worst crime took place when 1 found the school attic. I climbed through the hatch and up out onto the school roof. I did this in a school break time, and all eyes were on me. This brought the Headmistress out, in curiosity, which led me to duck behind a chimney, out of sight. Before retreating, I hung a pair of knickers on the flagpole.

Sadly, there was one other way I grabbed attention. Looking back it gives a sense of shame and remorse, but I would dream up various ailments. Perhaps real in my mind, I do not really know looking back. This always meant a trip to our doctor, and from there to a hospital specialist. I always hoped something may be found to be wrong. However, I was disappointed if things were not so, and they very rarely were, if ever.

I was doing well with my music. I passed my grade five theory with 98%. My teacher said she was so proud of me. I then passed my grade seven piano practical examination, and 1 entered my first piano playing competition, at the Stratford Music Festival. I played part of a sonata by Mozart. I gained 79% with good comments. This competition was the start of many more. It was at this point that my teacher said that I should consider taking music as a career. Looking back, I cannot help thinking that my life would have been very different, and may have been better. Who knows?

One day, at school, it was decided that berets need no longer be worn. As I was supposed to have my head covered when out, this was a bombshell for me. Other children in this religion often put on their hat, or whatever, when they left home, but took it off when out of sight of their parents. I wore my beret, because I had been told by my mother that God could see me without it. Looking back, I cannot help thinking that God would rather have seen me without my beret than listen to my awful lies as to why I was wearing a beret when questioned by the girls at school.

I sobered down in my last year, at school, and the Headmistress made me Head girl. I felt very proud, but my parents were not at all encouraging, or even seem bothered. I learnt that the Headmistress had told them on one occasion that this was her plan, simply to build up some confidence in me. I felt crushed, and all the glory of the position left me. It did not have any effect, as it was my religion that was sapping all my confidence.

Towards my 0 levels, as they were then called, my concentration seemed to leave me. I could not focus on the work they entailed. I do not know why this happened. I needed five passes, as I had decided that I wished to become a teacher, and move on to High school, and sixth form. I only passed three subjects, one of which was music. I had to stay on at the school, in order to at least pass two more. Fortunately I was able to do so. My days at this school were over, after eleven years of being a pupil there.

Progress is Made

The summer and Easter school holidays were spent with my grandparents at Ramsgate. We travelled around by bus or train and also did a fair amount of walking. Most of our time was spent on a sandy beach where I dipped in and out of the sea. As a child, I would plan my week, one day I would dig a hole, another day build a sand castle, and so on. This rigidity that was a pattern in my life was really quite unnecessary. On reflection, it would have a happier situation to have taken each day as it came and just enjoy myself doing whatever took my fancy at the time.

I loved the local swimming pool on the front at Ramsgate. It had sea water that came in with the tide, but I did hate the smelly, slimy changing cubicles. It was the largest pool I think I have ever seen, equipped with many diving boards and slides. It was not long before I had worked out how many lengths I needed to swim a mile. When I had achieved this I was as proud as if I had been swimming in the Olympics.

One very sad day, a day that will be with me for the rest of my life. I made my way to the pool on my own, to swim another mile. I was very engrossed as I swam the lengths, but after time I realised that I was the only one left in the pool, and when I climbed out I was aware that something awful had happened. A boy had fallen from a high diving board, hit his head on a concrete board coming down, and fallen unconscious into the very murky water to the bottom of the pool. The life guards were repeatedly diving down in an attempt to find him. When they finally pulled him from the water, he was dead. There was a deathly silence around the pool. He was the son of the man who ran the pool cafe, and he was in pieces, that poor man. I cannot remember any events that followed, only that I just went home and I too was in pieces. It was after this that they closed off the diving area at the pool.

On reflection, my grandparents must have gone to great expense to feed us while we were with them over the holidays. My grandfather had quite a good job by then, but they were given no financial help from us and I think this was very remiss of my parents. My granny and grandpa always gave me pocket money and other gifts when I was with them on holiday, they were so generous.

My father still had a violent temper that could erupt at any time and I found this very frightening. He would often start an argument at a meal time, especially with my grandparents. At home when I had gone to bed my father would then start arguing with my mother and I could hear him from my bedroom. It would often go on until about midnight. I was not very old when I started going downstairs purely to tell him to shut up, and I was also aware that he beat my mother. The next day my mother would show me all her bruises, and perhaps this was unwise, but it simply made me hate my father even more. On the other hand it made me cling to my mother, as I did not wish to even be with my father. One occasion when on holiday my father arranged for my brother and me to sail to France for the day. My brother went, but as usual I stayed with my mother, and this behaviour of mine went on sadly, until his death.

When I reached my mid teens I had grown out of going to my grandparents at Ramsgate every holiday. My father had a driving license which he had obtained before the driving test became compulsory, but to boost his confidence he took a few lessons at the wheel. We hired a car for the four of us and my grandparents. We went to south Devon, staying at a guest house, on a farm. It was a bit of a squeeze in the car, but we managed. Also the car had a radio, forbidden by our religion, but we were allowed to use at times, and that was great. We all enjoyed this holiday but it was the last time that we included our grandparents and I think they were sad about this.

We were always limited as to where we could go for holidays, because we had to be near one of our religious gatherings, and this really spoilt things for me because there was no escaping the Sundays that I still dreaded. It was one holiday that I discovered that there was a lady in our gathering who was a window cleaner, but to keep to the rules she had to wear a skirt, as trousers were not allowed in our religion. I will not comment further.

For many years I made my clothes, such as dresses, blouses and even coats and I also did a lot of knitting. Even today I still enjoy knitting, along with many other forms of craft. I may now have the television on but my hands are nearly always busy at the same time. The difference today is the rise of charity shops and these do put a stop to making certain clothes.

Also in my later teens I decided to breed budgerigars, and to do this I needed two aviaries, one of which I would use purely for breeding. A friend gave me one that he no longer used and the other I mostly built myself. I had picked up many carpentry tips from my grandfather and also my brother, so I think I had some skill in this direction, and also a lot of luck.

The completed aviary was a success, and it was soon populated with a good variety of budgies. However, it took my mother some time to come to terms with their raucous singing and chirping. I then purchased some nesting boxes for the other aviary, and selected pairs of birds, to hopefully breed. Each day I peeped into the boxes, until one day there were eggs. My anticipation and excitement was huge. Still I kept a daily vigil, until the day came when they had hatched. It brought home to me the wonder of creation. The little chicks were so tiny and fragile, and occasionally I had to clean them. These birds taught me so much. I was in awe as to the way the parent birds cared for their young. I continued breeding these birds for some time, and I did manage to sell some.

I also had an interest in Lepidoptera, that being butterflies and moths. My parents had taken me to a silk worm farm in Kent, and I came home with some eggs of a variety of moths and butterflies. I made them their boxes, and fitted them out with the correct leaves or plants .On one occasion I sent away for the eggs of the foreign moon moth. One day my mother and I had the privilege of watching it emerge from a cocoon unfolding its wet wings, until reaching its full size. A little like blowing up a balloon. I thought at the time that only God could do this, no man could make anything so perfect and glorious, with such a hue of colours.

The time had come for me to enter high school, or grammar school, for the sixth form. There were some girls there from my religion, so I had company in that sense, and I did fit in. I had also decided that 1 wanted to teach physical education at secondary level. I made the school hockey team, and I was due to take my grade eight final piano examination. Along with these I entered some royal life saving exams and finally obtained the silver award. This last exam was challenging, as I had to learn to swim feet first on my back, do various acrobats in the water, and finally I had to swim one mile, up and down the pool, fully dressed, including a pair of shoes. At the end of the swim I had to undress without touching the bottom of the pool. In other words, tread the water. What struck me with horror was the fact that I might have forgotten to put my swimming costume on first. I had put it on, so the examiner was spared his blushes. I also was made a member of the R.L.S.S. for one year. After the silver award there was a three- hour exam which if passed gave one the title after your name of R.L.S.S. I could have gained this award quite easily when at college, and I regret that I did not do so.

I managed to obtain eight 0' levels, not a great achievement, and it was the custom of the local education authority to put prospective teachers in for a teaching practice into a local school. I managed to do this, but I was scared of teaching girls so near my age and in many ways I was more comfortable in the classroom setting, rather than with physical education. Maybe I should have heeded this warning.

The Plymouth Brethren, my religious gathering, were beginning to invent more rules. It was decided, and I do not know why, that the children of this strange religion should be withdrawn from school assemblies. I found it painful and embarrassing asking the headmistress to release me from her assemblies, when I did not even know the reason why. Instead, all those of us in this sect had to sit in the school library, where those feeling extra holy decided we should have a Bible quiz. I only know that I would have preferred to attend the school's Christian assembly, which consisted of hymns, prayers and Bible readings. In some schools this regime caused much friction especially in private schools, and rightly so.

I had been going through the process of choosing colleges. Again, I had to choose a college where I could attend one of our religious gatherings. There was no escape. However, I chose and was selected for Avery Hill Teacher Training College in London to study Advanced Physical Education and a second subject of my choice. It was also the first year for teachers to train for three years instead of two.

Then my life came to an abrupt halt. I left school one afternoon and headed home to have something to eat. I then set off for my piano lesson. I was tearing down a steep hill; I could have been doing 20-30 mph, 1 may have hit a pot hole or something may have caught my front wheel. I do not know. A witness told me later that I went over the handle bars onto my face. I was taken to hospital; there was an awful lot of blood and my school uniform had to be cut from me. I do remember a doctor putting down his cigarette and stitching my head. I was in hospital for two weeks. The whole of my face was cut, and my nose broken 1 also had severe concussion. My first visitor was my piano teacher, who brought four peaches. I missed my piano exam, I missed a camping holiday and I also missed the sixth form leaving party.

Within our religious gathering, or meeting, there was one female, a Mrs Taylor, often called Brother Taylor for the way she was so bossy, and holy. While I was in hospital I had a long letter, not of sympathy, but stating how God had saved me from the wicked and unholy sixth form leaving party. My reaction to that was that in fact that I should have had a trailer behind my bike with all those attending the party of my religion. Not only that, she used to ride around on a bike wearing a tweed skirt, and of course some sort of hat. If on her travels she spied one of the female members without something on their head, she went to the length of writing and posting a long letter to that sinner about the fact that she had seen them without a head covering. If only she had known what I said and thought about her behind her back, which was no doubt an even greater sin than my uncovered head.

More and more rules were being laid down by this sect I was part of. We were no longer allowed to belong to any society or association. It was dubbed an unholy link, as we were included on a list with wicked people. It was agreed that nurses should have a cross by their names, and this made it O.K. for them, but how I do not know. Then it was ruled that no one was to be allowed to work on Sunday, simply because that person must attend the gathering, or meeting. This meant a serious loss of income to some members, but no help was ever offered to any in this situation. In fact, all these rules were being dreamt up by the leader of this sect. He was a Mr James Taylor, in fact an alcoholic, living in America. He was worshiped like a god, and had the nick name of Big Jim. I was so bothered, almost tormented as to where and how far these rules were going, and what impact they might have on my life. They were also seriously denting my confidence even further. As I was soon to start college I was being pressurised into becoming a Christian, so as to fit into the new gathering near my college. My mother had told me in the past that becoming a Christian would bring persecution so as I considered that I had enough of that anyway, then being a Christian was not an option at that time. In my new gathering I would have to qualify to take communion or, as we had to call it, breaking of bread, and I would be in serious trouble if I did not comply with the rules. So I did become a Christian but more in theory than in practice. I was then seen by a couple of men in my gathering and asked what I considered to be stupid questions, and I was not particularly truthful. I was asked if I belonged to any associations, I said no, but of course I did belong to the Royal Life Saving Society, but it was not an association.

In the first year at my college, students could be billeted out. It so happened that a lady in my religion did this, and it was arranged that I would be with her, along with another member also starting at the college. I did not like this arrangement in many ways, but there was nothing that I could do about it.

So my life was about to enter another phase, with the good, bad and indifferent.

College Life

Long before I started college I felt sad, and fearful at the thought of leaving home. My father had a means test, and it was agreed that I could have £3.00 a week. This was ample for my expenses while at college.

My mother accompanied me on the first day of college. Many first year students were billeted in the area and I was billeted, at my request, to a lady in my religion. There was also another student of my religion also with me. I did not like sharing a room, as I had never done this before. My land lady, Mrs Robbins, was a kindly person, and she had two young, lovely children, a boy called Michael, and a girl called Helen. Mrs Robbins had students each year for financial reasons. Early in her marriage her husband left for Australia with another woman. Mrs Robbins never quite got over the shock of this.

On that first day, my mother stayed for a light meal, but when she left to return home, I had an empty sick feeling in my stomach. Part of my life had gone. I had a sick feeling for about a week, as did many first year students.

There were four students of my religion at the college, and it was a foregone conclusion that we would keep together. As time went on I gradually began to break away from them, and so gain a sense of freedom, or perhaps rebellion.

Associations, in all forms, were of course forbidden to us, and this included college unions, something else I had to withdraw from. In fact this did not take place as I thought. On entering any college joining the union was automatic. I later learnt that many from my religion entered colleges and kept quiet over the issue of unions.

Why was I so anxious to try and adhere to the rules of my religion? I was scared about how all these ever increasing rules were going to affect my life, and the quality of it. I did not know then that this strange religion would eventually collapse and bring me such joy. If only I had known. It would have been something to look forward to, and encourage me to cling on.

The first few days were spent sorting out timetables and various interviews with lecturers. I was interviewed along with my fellow students and lecturers. Each student reported on all their sporting achievements. My confidence fell, until I remembered my Award of Merit in swimming. I went into this in some detail, stating that I gained full marks, and that this was the first time in thirty years that this had happened. This was reported to headquarters, with a view to me being used for demonstration purposes. My confidence soared, it had paid off. The lecturers were so impressed, and I was level pegging with all the other students.

I had decided to do music for my second subject, partly because my piano teacher at school was adamant that I should take up music for my career. This did not work out. I did not like my new piano teacher, and I found it difficult to fit in all the theory and practise in both subjects, the work load was massive. I was accepted into the art course, as my second subject, and I just enjoyed myself. I went to lectures only if 1 felt like doing so, yet I worked hard at the subject, doing what I felt like doing in my own time. I covered many aspects of art, passing top with distinction in my final year.

I was auditioned and accepted into the college choir. We practised on Monday evenings, with an interval for supper. This did coincide with the prayer meeting of my religion, but I was not censored. Perhaps they prayed for my waywardness, if they did, it had no effect.

I studied for my Amateur Swimming Association Teachers certificate for swimming and diving. I was the only student to pass these two exams.

Towards the end of my first year, after a gymnastic lecture, the lecturer weighed each student. This spelt disaster for me, as I was told to lose a few pounds. This hit me hard. Those few pounds I interpreted as stones. This was the exact date of the anorexia nervosa that plagued me so cruelly, for so many years. From that day, the crash dieting led me to constantly think of food, and all the things I would love to eat. I set myself a target weight, with the thought that when I achieved it then I could eat normally. When I reached that weight, then I lowered the target, and so it went on. I was never slim enough in my eyes. I craved the cakes I saw in the cake shops, and hot meals I saw and smelt in the college canteen, and I could only have salads. I could be so hungry, tired and miserable and my periods stopped for a very long time. There were times when hunger drove me to binge and

I would eat until I felt ill. Then I started taking laxatives, thinking I was losing weight, in fact I was only losing body fluids, and this was very temporary.

In my second year at college my weight crept up a few pounds, and a lecturer noticed this and pulled me to one side and asked me about my weight. I do not remember my reply but I did have tears in a quiet place. How I envied that student who when asked about her weight replied that it was absolutely fine and just laughed at the lecturer.

Beneath it all I was tough, and I had to be. I came second in my college in a fitness test that was organised by a body of people who were aiming to compare the fitness of physical education students in other countries. The Swiss came top in fitness. I did quite well in sport. I belonged to the cricket team, and also the lacrosse team. One Saturday we had a lacrosse match against Dartford Physical Education College. It was raining, the pitch was sheer mud. On our way back to the changing rooms, by luck we passed their indoor swimming pool. We all went in stripped of our kit and had a swim in the nude. We called it our stolen swim.

As part of our teacher training we all had to have teaching experience in schools. My lack of self confidence hindered my ability in the classroom. I was afraid that problems might arise that would be out of my depth to control. This never happened at any time in my career as a teacher, although one headmistress told me that I was too strict and I replied that I would not change my approach to discipline. My first teaching practice took place in a primary school. The children were having a craft lesson making all sorts of little novelties. I asked one young boy what he was making. Of course I should have known. He very indignantly told me he was making a horse, and gave me a withering look that told me I should have known. I then made matters worse by saying that horses did not have five legs. He then slowly counted each leg and triumphantly declared that the fifth was a widdler. As this was longer than the legs it meant that I had to spend some time gazing out of the window to compose myself.

One lesson I was reading a primary class a story. They were sitting around my chair, all very cosy. They were quiet, therefore I assumed they were engrossed with the story, and I was happy that it was going well. That is, until a hand shot up and promptly asked me how old I was. From then on I assumed I was reading to myself, leaving them to ponder my age my first name, and so on.

Another big mistake took place in a dreadful comprehensive school, feared by many. I had to take a class of fourteen year old pupils for a music lesson. I told them we would learn the Ash Grove song. I immediately knew my error when they all burst into song,

"0 you are a bunion
With a face like a pickled onion
A nose like a squashed tomato and ears like corned beef."

They didn't get very far into the song when I hit the piano keys and threatened them that it would be fine by me if we sat until midnight to get the correct words. I did succeed but if I had backed down in any way I knew there could have been discipline problems.

In my second year at college the lecturers arranged for us to go to Wales on an outward bound course. This would involve sailing, canoeing, pot holing and hiking. How I longed to be able to go, but because of so many rules in my religion, it was out of bounds for me. I felt so stupid telling the lecturer in charge why I could not go, making excuses that even seemed stupid to me.

In my second year at college I should have been going into residence, as was the custom. I would have liked to have done this, but it would have thrown up all sorts of religious problems. Instead I had to brace myself to go before the college Principal to ask permission to spend another year with my landlady Mrs Robbins. She did grant this after she had tied me up in knots and reduced me to tears. After all if she thought it was stupid, then so did I.

The Witch's Haunt

The women in this religion were not allowed to cut their hair. Then the time came when it was decided that their hair was in fact their glory. This meant that young and old had to have their long locks flowing loose. It could no longer be neatly tied up on their heads.

Then the women had to swop their hats for a humble, a rather scruffy headscarf. Looking round the religious gathering with wisps of hair sticking out under a scarf it did indeed look like a witch's haunt.

Mr James Taylor, the leader of this regime, could do or say nothing wrong. The saints declared him as being holy. He would take a so called service with a glass of whisky at his feet. He could be the worse for drink and repeat the same phrase for nearly an hour. If he took another man's wife this was looked upon as an honour. He was also heard to say in a service that women's boobs were lovely.

I hated him and dreaded what rule he might come out with next, each time fuelled by the spirits that fired him onward. His rules were ludicrous, as though he had me in his clasp and there was no way of escape.

No one was allowed to vote. The saints said that God chose the government. How I do not know. At an early age I saw the stupidity of this notion. I tried to explain to my mother that if we prayed as to who we should vote for then the right government would be elected. At any time my mother felt cornered she just told me not to be silly.

The saints then decided that all their so called churches should not have any windows. Perhaps they were afraid of peeping toms spying on the evil that went on inside. All these churches took on the appearance of a gas chamber. There was plenty of gas inside.

The times of the Sunday gatherings took on ridiculous dimension. The first service started at five a.m. and the other services followed at three hourly intervals. Somehow this was supposed to follow the pattern of the resurrection. More likely it followed someone's lively imagination. I usually caught up on some shut eye in the service.

These saints were adamant that the world would come to an end on a Sunday. I could only dream as to how this would work in other countries through the world.

Where we lived and how we lived was dictated. We had to live in detached houses. Being connected by bricks and mortar to our neighbours would amount to an unholy link. Then some bright spark went even further. The drains were linked to our neighbours. Perhaps this was an unclean link. So all the faithful ones now had to have cesspits. I only hope the neighbours were not connected with any unsavoury odours.

School children of these saints had to withdraw from various activities that might warp their minds. Two young pupils told their teacher that they could not attend the cinema outing as they were children of the saints. The teacher retorted that they were more likely children of devils.

Should one of the saints put a foot wrong but not to the extent that necessitated their being thrown out of the congregation, then they were shut up. This meant they had to sit at the back of all gatherings and were consequently ostracized. They were half in and half out.

To top up the congregations all aspiring young mothers were expected to produce a baby each year. They certainly bred like rabbits.

The next rule was not far behind. Because Jesus was a carpenter and worked with His hands, this meant that all the men in the congregation now had to work with their hands. They had to give up jobs and do just that. A dentist was allowed to carry on as he did work with his hands. Perhaps the saints had free fillings and so on. One young man with cystic fibrosis was put to work on a building site. This was just plain stupid, extremely unfair and even cruel. That is what these people stooped to all in the name of religion. The women were not allowed to work. They just stayed home and had babies.

It goes without saying that all marriages had to take place within the religious gathering.

Appearance and dress took on a further slant. All the males, if they had any hair, were obliged to have it cut short back and sides. On the other hand, any whiskers below the hair line, such as moustaches and beards, had to disappear.

Then their wardrobe came under fire. No more ties. Their shirts had to be blue, because they said it was a heavenly colour. This was their uniform.

The women also had to adhere to a dress code. Denim skirts had to be worn at all times. Their long locks, or glory, flowed loose, topped with a skimpy headscarf. It looked more like a handkerchief. This was accompanied with a facial expression of despair and resignation. One could always pick them out in a crowd. Any head covering had to be worn all day, possibly in case they had to urge to pray. Even school children wore these scarves to school, but ripped them off at the school gates.

I can only assume that the saints of this strange religion were possessed with a vivid imagination, possibly fuelled by the spirits they consumed.

This set- up was beginning to show cracks. Those who followed the leader with enthusiasm and alcohol to excess, the spirits of many youngsters took a different twist. This caused much amusement to the rebels, including me.

One man tried to take a so called service and was drunk. He repeated the line of a song for nearly an hour. Many youngsters had to leave the room, convulsed with hysterics. The rest of us were giggling, except his mother whose face was scarlet with embarrassment. Another service we sat for an hour waiting for the saint to come and deliver his words of wisdom. I cannot imagine what words he was coming out with, as he had been deliberately locked in a toilet for the hour.

These youngsters were never short of mischief. They sat at the back of any congregation, with an air of innocence. They had their Bibles on their laps, often with a novel on top. Sometimes they made toast with cigarette lighters. One night they crept into the basement and plunged us all into darkness. On one occasion we all turned up to find the hall filled with hydrogen balloons hanging from the ceiling. During services there was often much heckling towards the faithful ones when they tried to take part.

In my third year we had to specialise in two subjects at advanced level. My obvious first subject was swimming. I wanted to take as my second subject, movement to music, a form of dance. As I could not have a record player like other students, I was at a disadvantage. I was in the dog house with the dance lecturer, because I opted for gymnastics as my second subject.

The biggest downside of my college life was this very strange religion, which I hated deep down. There were three meetings on Sunday; these local and in walking distance. In the week we had to travel several miles to a meeting, either in a mini coach driven by one of the saints, or by public transport. There were times when I did not get home until gone midnight.

Our religion told us to live separate lives to anyone not in our religion. We were not allowed to sit and eat with anyone not in our religion. This divided families, meaning that a daughter could not eat with her mother if she was not a member. If this rule, or any rule was broken and it came to light, then that sinner was thrown out of the religion. The student living with us made it clear that she did not agree with this rule, so she was duly thrown out of our church and also the billet, and therefore had to move into college halls of residence, as she was not allowed to sit and eat with us.

All eating places such as cafes or restaurants were out of bounds to us. I do not know why as we were allowed to eat on buses and trains.

Alcohol flowed freely among the saints, no doubt as a fuel to keep them going. It was drunk to excess. There was one chap amongst us who worked for Thames Water, and they became very concerned about his excessive drinking. I assume that was alcohol.

Now Mrs Robbins could no longer take in students and this meant that she could no longer make ends meet financially, but our church did not come forward with any assistance. Those outside our religion were labeled as being unclean. Along came the next rule; we were not allowed to have pets as animals were also unclean. They are God's creatures, and what He made is perfect.

Verses were taken out of context in the Bible. "The solitary are put into families" now meant that no one could live alone. Consequently anyone living alone was promptly thrown into a household. Then some bright spark happened to read in his Bible that, "Ants are a working people". He then assumed that they obviously didn't have holidays. So because of these wretched ants no one in our religion was now allowed to have a holiday.

Then to my horror someone ferreted out the words, "Leave home to get married". As I had left home to go to college, I was told just that." "Go home". My mind was made up. I was not going home in my final year. I planned to buy a motor bike and travel backwards and forwards. I was scared, but I did just that.

With the help of my brother I purchased a second hand 250cc motor bike. It was big and very heavy, and I was scared, but I did cope with it. The journey from my home to college was nearly twenty miles. I had to use the Woolwich ferry to cross the river Thames. At times, I had to queue as the bridges were up to let passing boats through, and this could take some time. I had to queue again to board the ferry, and then negotiate my way onto the ferry. On a cold day I would relish the heat of the engine room. Sometimes a blanket of fog would render the ferry out of action. This meant I had to use Blackwall Tunnel on my way to college, and it was horrendous. There were tankers and other large vehicles, making me look very small indeed. There was noise and fumes, and we just crawled through that tunnel. I could not even hear the engine of my bike. I was in a very dark place, in more ways than one. On my return home very late one night the tunnel was mine, and I shot through it at seventy miles an hour which was about the limit of the bike's power. This earned me the title of tearaway, which I hold and am reminded of to this very day. In a sneaky way I am quite proud of it.

There were some days, when the weather was fine, that I did the journey on my push bike. In the back of my mind I expect I had the idea that I might get my weight down. Occasionally I made the journey by train, but whatever method of transport I chose, it always seemed a long trek, very tiring and I felt all the time that I was fighting a losing battle. At the same time my studies did not suffer, hard as it was at times. Although I had to keep putting the correct amount of fuel in the bike, I am afraid that I did not put the correct amount of fuel in me. This did not help matters

If the weather was bad, Mrs Robbins gave me a room to call my own, and I would stay with her. This was very gracious of her and a big help for me.

They say variety is the spice of life. This strange religion, or sect, certainly provided us with that. I began to attend the so called services expecting to be entertained with whatever these youngsters may provide for me. This alone kept me going. There was no spiritual food as one should expect from a church.

It was this demise that eventually brought the collapse of this strange religion. This was a relief for me as some normality began to creep in. I will cover this in a later chapter.

I Start Teaching

I passed my Teachers Certificate of Education, and I was top in my year. I achieved merit in advanced physical education, my first subject, and distinction for art, my second subject.

I started teaching in a secondary modern school for girls. I taught physical education and human biology at G.C.E. '0' level, as it was known as then.

It is said that teachers are born and not made, and basically I knew that I was in that category. However, because of my past I still lacked self confidence and felt unable to achieve what was required of me. In many ways this had a crippling effect on me. I was still desperately trying to lose weight. I weighed myself daily and kept a diary of everything that I ate. I was always hungry and weary. Although I was teaching a physically demanding subject I looked upon it as a means of losing weight. Life was tough. Also, I had been privately educated and it was a shock when I started teaching in a council run school. There was a roughness there and uniform was not enforced.

The school was divided between the boys and girls with a head teacher for each school. To begin with I was in charge of a first year class and managed to learn the names of the 450 girls in the school. Despite my own problems I gave my best to my profession as was expected of me.

My background and upbringing had taught me something that college did not teach me. I was able to empathise with the pupils and how they ticked. I could feel for them in their problems and be there for them. I had an intuitive sense of compassion when needed.

Frances was my first casualty. She was sitting at the back of the class looking sad and tearful. I learnt that her father had permanently left the home. Frances was devastated and on sedatives. At no time would she leave the classroom, as in break time or dinner time. At these times I would grab my coffee from the staffroom and head down to Frances. I would gently coax her to come into the playground with me where I would find some girls from her class to take her into their group and they were always willing to do this. I did take the opportunity to explain to the class, in her absence, the reason she needed extra kindness and care. This was a tactic that I used in teaching as it helped overcome bullying.

Frances sought me out one morning in floods of tears. I thought something dreadful had taken place. In fact she had just spoilt the first page of her new French exercise book. Of course we all liked to start a new exercise book neatly and hopefully keep it that way. I simply solved the problem by giving her a new exercise book from the stock cupboard, then solved her next problem as to what she should do with the old one. I told her that she could use it for drawing, but added that she told no one as I did not want the whole school coming to me for a new exercise book.

My Christian faith led me tentatively say to her that there was a Father in Heaven she could talk to and ask for help, and that I did at times.

All this went home to Mum as each Christmas I received a lovely bouquet of flowers. I was thankful, but was sad when staff said that it was not my problem and why did I bother. Teaching, to me, did not start at nine and finish at four.

There was the lighter side. On one occasion a master sent another master a large box taped and tied. When undone it was found to be empty. The box was duly returned and filled with coal from the coal shed. However this time the box remained unopened and left on the master's desk. Some of these coals happened to be hot, and overnight they burnt through the desk and through the floor. The next morning the fire engines took care of the situation, while the headmaster just told the masters not to be so stupid in future. Perhaps he saw the funny side of the prank to take it so lightly.

The headmaster had an allotment which he tended before school. He would take school assembly dressed in his flowing gown, but still with his very muddy boots. It looked somewhat ridiculous.

In my second year of teaching I was promoted to head of department for physical education. Along with the department and staff to organise there was also the field and swimming sports days. I took part in a staff swimming race one year. I was still in my twentieth year when a girl in my class came to me and said. "Miss you aint harf a good swimmer, well that's as seeing you're middle aged." I cannot remember my answer, but she did come to me again and said. "Miss was that one of the things that you really shouldn't say". I said that I did not mind what she said to me, but to be careful what she said to other people.

As I have mentioned, I taught human biology to exam level. The girls I taught were known in those days as eleven plus failures, and their teaching had to be extremely thorough. Such as the time when I taught the rib cage in the body and I asked them to draw a rough diagram of the rib cage, where it started and where it ended. One girl's rib cage started at under the chin and ended at her ankles. I asked her to stand and look at her ankles, and asked if she had any ribs down there, so problem solved.

In those days they had to write quite lengthy essays and the spelling had to be correct. It was not accepted to spell the Eustachian tube in the ear as Euston station. Not as seems today, tick the right answer on a form, and as long as the examiner knows what the pupil means, then that's good enough.

We did not teach sex in those days but rather human reproduction. I started with the reproduction of the amoeba, the frog, then quite naturally to that of the human being.

I was pleased to manage a pass rate each year of about twenty girls out of about twenty two.

We had a foreign teacher at the school, who did not have a good command of English. The girls in her lessons were very forthcoming in extending her vocabulary. Unfortunately they were not always words to be found in the English dictionary.

After a few years the two schools merged with one head teacher in control, and new buildings were added. At this point I moved into the new art rooms to teach art and craft.

One of my first classes was fourteen year old boys who had been sent from another school. Like hooligans, their feet and bags soon rearranged everything in the room and they were also very vocal.

I banged my table and screamed that they put the room straight. When this was done I told them that it was obvious that they didn't want a lesson, and what was more I didn't feel like giving them one. As a result, I made them spend the rest of the lesson with their hands on their heads. Any pleas that their arms were aching and so on, I responded with the word, "Tough". However, they turned out to be one my best examination classes.

Near my art room was a small cupboard, in which pupils smoked by candle light. On one occasion they left and a candle had fallen, unknown to them, and this partially gutted the new science block. A fleet of fire engines took care of the situation, along with much excitement from the onlookers.

One or two staff, including me, took a party of senior boys on a tour round London. I nobly volunteered to escort them up the Monument to point out the famous buildings on the horizon. Unlike me they had no difficulty clambering up a hundred or so stairs. On reaching the summit they were only interested in one thing. That was spitting over the railings, and enquiring of me as to whether their spit would reach the ground. I felt like throwing them over the railings for being so ungrateful.

I witnessed the first teachers' strike. In the school only two of us refused to strike, including me, and the pupils for those teachers could voluntarily come to their lessons. Every lesson I had pupils, and it was during one of these lessons that a boy said to me, "Those teachers what have gone on strike, they teach for the money, but you teach because you want to teach. When those teachers on strike come back we're going to give em hell". "They did just that by going on strike over their home work and a lot more besides.

One afternoon I arrived home from school to find my father was expecting an ambulance as he was experiencing chest pains. After a long wait I drove him, as well as my mother, to the hospital. They admitted him onto the cardiac ward as his condition was serious, and I think he realised that he was nearing his end. At this point he apologised for his sexual behaviour with me. It was hard to think of all those girls he could not apologise to, but I did forgive him for myself, although it was hard. He died early the next morning following a heart attack at the age of sixty. That chapter of my life, with the trauma from my father, was now over.

I had a minor accident on my motor bike, and this led me to buy my first second hand car. After lessons I passed the test on the second attempt. I enjoyed driving and I then had further lessons with a view to taking the Institute of Advanced Motorist test. The test was horrendous. I had to drive for two hours in every road condition. There were busy roundabouts, congested country lanes and main roads where I was told to overtake. In the most congested road conditions, the examiner would ask me what the road sign was that we had just passed. On each occasion I managed to make a correct guess. I did pass the test.

I resumed my piano lessons, with a view to taking my grade eight that I had been unable to take owing to my cycle accident. I took the test one bitterly cold day in winter. The heating in the place had ceased working, the examiner was dressed for arctic conditions, and my fingers felt like icicles. Somehow I managed to pass the exam.

After my father's death my mother and I moved into a smaller house. Soon after this my eating disorder led to me being hospitalized. I was in fact there for five months I was injected with insulin at one point, which meant that if I did not eat sufficiently- I would lapse into a coma which made me feel like death. During these five months my mother came to see me every day. There were days when I was so depressed I didn't even speak to her. Her journey involved two separate buses. That is a mother's love. My stay in that hospital was not without incidence. At one point I smashed my head open on a wall, which necessitated stitches. I took an overdose in rebellion because they didn't overcome my sleepless nights. I was not allowed out of the building, so at night after plumping up my bed I climbed out of a window. All this was done in rebellion over something, with some success. After all this I left the hospital still with my eating disorder. It ended suddenly many years later. I did have follow up help from a psychiatrist after leaving the hospital. She said to me that she did not go by the book, and she certainly did not. To start with she told the most awful lies, which I did not see through until sometime later. She came and stayed with me for a week, while my mother went on holiday. We went out for evenings with her boyfriend, and one night while at a Greek night club she became drunk. We were driven home, where I insisted that her boyfriend helped undress her, and also leave his telephone number.

One time we took a picnic to a park and she took a photo of me, and I took one of her. This proved to be her undoing. When I realised that my treatment was far from ethical and was in fact having a detrimental effect on me, I wrote to the head of the psychiatric department, including a photo of her by the picnic basket.

She was duly severely disciplined, and other arrangements were made for me.

There were times when I became so guilty after having eaten what to me was too much, that it wasn't long before I started making myself sick. This meant I was now bulimic, and this was worse than the anorexia, because now I was out of control. Every meal and every mouthful was doomed to go down the pan. I could no longer enjoy food because of the consequences of eating. I would have frequent binges followed by sickness, and repeat the whole thing again and again. I was so unhappy. At times I would claim that this was my last time and then I would be in control. I said this many times. However a day came when I was faced with a large quantity of food that I had purchased. That was the day that my eating disorder left me for good. I looked at the food in disgust and said out loud to myself, "I cannot do this ever again." To this day I have never looked back, I can now eat and enjoy.

My piano teacher began placing me in piano competitions, with some success. My highest award was a gold medal, and first place in a competition, playing a Beethoven sonata.

I began giving piano lessons at home, and also accompanied on the piano for school concerts, and sometimes school assembly. My love of art and craft encouraged me to go to various classes, and I often made my own gifts. Sometimes I would sell some of my craft work. I was also able to make many of my own clothes as I was adept at needlework, knitting, and crochet. After a time my mother and I downsized house again, and this is the home that I live in today. The house and garden are just the right size for me to look after, and take much pleasure in.

After some time I moved to another girl's school, in a very poor part of London. I was still teaching art and craft and eventually became head of department. There was never a dull moment in this school, and I cannot elaborate on them all.

We had our first bomb alert. It was possible that one of the pupils had made the phone call, but we had to take it seriously. In those days bomb alerts were almost unheard of. The girls were lined up in the playground, and the police duly arrived. They set about playing ball with the girls and told us teachers to look around our classrooms in search of the bomb. I paced twice round my classroom, without opening any cupboards, and reported back that I had not found any bombs. It was the next day, while sitting in the staff room, that we realised what mutts we had been. That in future the police would hunt for bombs.

We did use the cane at school, mainly for bullying, and as a result we did not have this problem at school. The harm a bully can do to an individual is far greater than a few taps from a stick on their hands. The very thought of the cane is the deterrent to an aspiring bully, and they are usually cowards anyway.

Many of the girls were extremely disruptive during the dinner break. They caused mayhem in the shops and tampered with the lifts in the flats. There were so many complaints that we decided to padlock the gates and contain them in the playground, or more to the point, the yard.

I introduced the bronze medal for the Duke of Edinburgh award. The girls had to pass a first aid text, and also plan a walk covering several miles. This meant working out bus and train times and a map to negotiate their trek. I always gave them my phone number, and on one occasion I sat in my car for a very long time. I was anxious, but I headed home. I then received a phone call from one of the girls, explaining that they had forgotten their map and had tried to guess the walk without it. They did not forget their lunch of course, but they did fail the test. The other venture for the girls was to give a party. This could be, for example, some O.A.P.s or children. This sometimes proved a challenge for me, as on one occasion the girls had chosen to give a party to some elderly people from a retirement home. I told two girls to buy some loaves of bread to make sandwiches, and I gave them money. However, they came back with a very large tub of ice cream. They thought the old ladies would much rather eat ice cream than sandwiches. I was annoyed and replied that in fact it was them that wanted the ice cream, and added that as there no freezers in the school the elderly people would be drinking the ice cream. On my second attempt they did come back with the loaves of bread. In the mean time I took the ice cream into the staff room, where we had a spoon each, and it was as though Christmas had come, and was very much enjoyed by all. I did not tell those girls.

One afternoon, an older girl was very distraught and admitted to having taken an overdose of tablets, and this proved to be genuine. She was taken to hospital in an ambulance. On her return, she was seen in the playground surrounded by all her cronies. It turned out that she gave a glowing account of her experience in hospital. That in fact it was just like a hotel. She had clean white sheets, no doubt unheard of in that part of London, and what was more she had her breakfast in bed. After this, there were quite a few girls who announced that they had taken an overdose, not that we really believed this, but it was a ruse to experience what seemed to them a life of luxury. This game was brought to an abrupt end when the head teacher promised the next girl who did this with dire consequences.

One afternoon I was driving through some local woods, when it was obvious that some police were removing a body. When I read the local newspaper I learnt that it was the father of one of the girls in the school. He had murdered his brother in law. My heart went out to this girl as I knew how she must be feeling. She was a bright girl, whose ambition was to become a doctor. She was also diabetic. However, at this point she gave up on herself, and started coming to school having eaten so many sweets that when she arrived at school she soon fell into a coma. This meant she had to be taken to hospital, and then the process was repeated. I wished to help her. I began speaking with her, to the effect that she was the important one, and although she could not forget what happened, she herself had done nothing wrong. That it was so important that she lived for herself and for her future and no one else. I coaxed her into working for the first aid test, which she passed. She was also very good at art work, so I placed her in some competitions, in which she did quite well. So her confidence grew and she began to believe in herself, and the induced comas ended.

The head teacher asked me to take a girl into my care. She was losing weight and tending to faint in assembly. It was quite common for parents to give their children money to buy their own food for the day. I asked Debbie why she was not buying herself food and she replied that she was saving up for a radio with the money. I explained that she would not get that radio because if she did not eat she would drop down dead. This really shook her. Consequently, each dinner break I took her to the shops and taught her how to spend her money on the food she needed for good health. This included a treat, such as potato crisps, and some money was put aside for her radio. We returned to school and had our lunch together in my classroom. We were soon able to buy a little radio, which did not cost as much as she anticipated. At the same time Debbie put on weight and became fit and well. For this, I was happy to have sacrificed my dinner break, which I would normally have spent in the staffroom, chatting and with my feet up.

We always had a hard core of girls playing truant; it was part of school life. There was one group that lightened their day by spending it on a tube train going round and round on the circle line. I can only think it would have been more interesting in school but the thrill of rebelling would not have been included. One day the head teacher promised this group that if they all stayed in school for one week; they could choose their teacher for that week. They chose me, and I was not happy. Their attention span was very poor and whatever task I gave them to work on, their hands would shoot up simultaneously. "Miss, we've finished". Their language and dress was no example to the youngest pupils. Deep down I would have preferred them to play truant. It was one of my worst weeks, and I begged the head teacher to spare me that in future.

Near the school there was a council home for teenage girls. When they did attend school they invariably had different colour hair each time. We used to tease them about this. Their truanting became so bad that eventually the police took it on themselves to escort them to school each morning. They dutifully delivered the girls through the front entrance, but the girls disappeared from the back of the building to their freedom.

I will end this chapter on what to me was a remarkable incident in my teaching career and gave me much cheer.

Paula was one of the most disruptive girls I had known. She had to be withdrawn from many lessons because the teachers could not control her behaviour. She did come to my lessons, but I was very uncomfortable, and felt as though I had a ticking time bomb in the room. One morning a group of Christians visited the school, and handed each girl a Bible. Paula was due to come to me for the first lesson of the day, but fifteen minutes into the lesson she had not appeared. I was getting very concerned, and was wondering what she was up to. Eventually she appeared, sauntering down the corridor absolutely absorbed with her Bible. My emotions at that point were mixed, as I was not expecting that turn of events from her. She calmly approached me with a little grin, and although I knew, I asked what she was reading. "A Bible, Miss, and it's about God and I believe it's all true". A little thrill of hope went through me, and I asked her if she would like to spend the lesson reading her Bible to which she replied, "Oh thank you, Miss". During the lesson some girls heckled her as to why she was not doing the lesson. I was about to speak for her, however, Paula spun round and explained that she was reading her Bible which was about God and it was all true. At the end of the lesson I held her back and simply said, "Well Paula?" With a bright face, she said," Miss I believe, I'm a Christian now, and I can't be naughty anymore." What a thrill! I had a chat with her and explained that it may not always be easy, and this was something that she would have to do herself, but that I would be in this classroom and any problems or upsets come straight to me and I would try and help. I prayed briefly with her, and told her how to pray. Several weeks went by when a teacher in the staffroom at morning break said. "What has happened to Paula? She has turned over a new leaf." Other staff heartedly agreed with this. Up to this point I had kept quiet about Paula because I knew that I had to allow her time to do this. Of course I spoke to her when I passed her in school. "Morning, Miss," she would say. Usually her Bible was visible in her bag. Now was the time to tell the staff that she had been reading a Bible given to her. That in doing so she had become a Christian and had realized that this meant she could no longer be naughty. Then I went on to say how becoming a Christian can give hope and turn a life around. There was a long silence in the room. Later, I told Puala that I thought she must have been special to God, that being of course the one and only God, as she was given that Bible on a day when she had me for the first lesson and was able to read it and become a Christian. Had it been a different lesson and teacher, she may have been told to put it away, and the opportunity lost. With our God nothing happens by chance, and we see this in His creation of the world around us.

My Freedom

Many steps and leaps took place before the unfolding of my life of freedom. My life has been a continuous learning curve. At times I do say, "If only". However, the past has gone and it is better to enjoy today, because it only comes once.

Eventually I retired from teaching with mixed feelings, and I often say that if I had my time again I would still work with young people. I enjoy their company and have a rapport with them.

I decided to sell my car, it was a wrench, but I have shops, buses and trains all nearby, and I knew that I would save myself the expense of running a car. Also, I would benefit from walking.

The strict religion that had plagued my life for so long collapsed. The leader, Mr James Taylor, was found in bed with a married woman. His devoted followers still maintained that he was holy and could do no wrong. The rest of the congregation declared, rightly, that it was adultery. After a set to one evening between the two sides, the devoted followers marched out of the building, taking all their ridiculous rules and regulations with them. They left behind a huge sigh of relief from the rest of us.

I now looked forward to a more normal life. At first my mother, after all these years, was very unsure as to which rules it was right to release. This was understandable, although I didn't think so at the time.

When I first visited the hairdresser, I came away with a hairstyle that any film star would have been proud of. In fact on my way home I experienced my first wolf whistle from a bunch of workmen. I was brought down to earth on arriving home by my mother's look of horror, and the words, "I thought you would come home looking extremely worldly." I had thrown all modesty aside, which was just what I had intended to do.

It was not long before I bought my first pair of trousers. I was so chuffed with them that I wore them most of the time. I wanted the whole world to see me emerging from the cocoon that I had been hiding in all my life.

After time my mother agreed to having a television. However, it had to be in a cabinet. The reason for this was, that if any of her friends from the church did not approve of this step in relaxing the rules, they couldn't see it. The fact that nothing is hidden from God didn't seem relevant.

I had my first cat, and to date, I have never been without one. I have always had a rescue cat, one that is in need of loving tender care and a home. At the time of writing I have a large black and white boy, who is now seventeen years old. He is my shadow, very bossy, and I love him dearly. I look upon him as one of God's creatures, and in fact I love all His creatures, and I get very upset when harm comes their way.

I am a born again believer. I put my faith and trust in God the Father, and His Son, Jesus Christ, who died for our sins on the cross. In asking Him for forgiveness of my sins, I know that when He returns to earth for His Christians, I will be taken up into Heaven, to live forever in a life of perfection and happiness. I must add here, that everyone must make a decision. Those who simply ask Jesus for their sins to be forgiven will have their place in Heaven. Those, on the other hand, who choose to reject this opportunity, and turn their backs on Christianity, will go to the alternative place, which is Hell. This will mean living forever in a dark and dreadful place, with no escape.

I had always been keen in photography, and I used both still and cine cameras. I put this to good use as I started travelling for the first time with touring companies. I also boarded a plane for the first time. As a child I had always dreamt of going to Switzerland and seeing all the snow. It was such a thrill to visit the Jungfrau in that country. The revolving restaurant in the snow covered mountain peaks, and the glorious ice caves. My time in Yugoslavia was special, and quite different. I spent time rowing a boat on the expansive Bala Lake. I had such a sense of peace in the lapping of the water and the solitude. I also swam in the cool refreshing water. I travelled by train through the massive caves in that country. I saw the dancing horses in a parade. Along with all this the scenery was breathtaking.

One holiday in Scotland, I stayed in a Christian hotel. Everyone, including the staff, was a Christian, and as a result there were no locks on the bedroom doors. We all felt perfectly safe, and to me it had a heavenly touch, with a sense of freedom.

There was a time when I looked for a new challenge, and embarked on ice skating. I managed to pass my grade two test. However the ice was solid and my frequent falls were painful, therefore this activity soon came to a halt.

I then turned to cycling, which turned out to be a pleasurable activity. I bought a racing bike, and enjoyed cycling, and also walking and swimming.

I was reminded of my teaching days one morning. I walked into my accountant's office, where I was greeted by the receptionist with the word's, "Hello Miss." It took the wind out of my sails, and I became "Miss". I asked her how she was getting on, and wished her all the best. The way I spoke made me feel an utter fool, as I was not at ease.

My mother was experiencing health problems in her advancing years. She had always been very controlling towards me. Therefore when she went into sheltered accommodation, I had an overwhelming sense of freedom. I did not have a sense of guilt, as I felt this freedom was owing to me: My life was now mine, and I very quickly began to put my stamp on my home and garden.

Today

My home has been decorated and furnished to my taste. I do not like clutter and ornaments, so those are kept to a minimum. I am not a hoarder, as my dear grandmother used to say. "If you haven't used a thing for two years, then you probably never will."

I love tending my garden. It is like painting a picture. It requires balance in height, texture and colour. It has to be pleasing to the eye. Now I am aiming for the tropical style of gardening, with bananas, palms, tree ferns and such like. It is so far successful and pleasing. I have a small summer house which I have furnished, and call my den. I have a large fish pond, and also space set aside for a hammock and sun lounger.

One year 1 had an open garden event for the public, and also had a picture of part of my garden in the local paper.

On my sixtieth and seventieth birthdays I filled my home with around twenty five friends, and had an outside caterer to lay on a lavish meal. Sadly, it was about this time that my mother passed away.

One year I did a sponsored swim for a local charity. I swam 106 lengths in a 25 metre pool, and raised £460 pounds. I think this amount was raised because no one expected me to swim quite that number of lengths. One generous donor anonymously put £106 through my letter box, with a note saying a quid a length.

I have joined a private health club for swimming, and to date I swim 30 lengths in around thirty five minutes. I swim all the strokes including butterfly, and in most strokes I swim arms and legs individually, using a float. The surroundings at the club are luxurious and I treat myself to one of their healthy meals.

One year I joined the Epping Forest local college and undertook a study in computer techniques, and therefore gained my certificates in IT. I am quite at home with my computer, and do not know how I would manage without it. Art and craft still ranks high on my agenda. I knit complicated patterns. At times I make jewellry, and I make all my birthday and Christmas cards. I also enjoy painting.

I always have the company of a cat, and have introduced a tropical aquarium. It is so relaxing watching the fish lazily swimming around.

Sometimes I wonder how I fit everything in to my days, because music is a passion of mine. I still play my piano for about an hour most days. Along with this I am learning to play the flute and also the violin. The violin is a real challenge for me. Occasionally I play in a local concert. I have a faith to help me in my life, and I enjoy attending my local church. I do not have the desire now to travel abroad, partly because I do not wish to fly now. It seems so unnatural for a lump of metal to fly up in the air, and if in a plane I would wonder what is keeping it up. So I travel around the U.K. with touring coaches, or by train to seaside resorts, or holidays with friends. All this as funds allow.

I am never bored, and never lonely. I have many friends, and I find it easy to chat to young and old, whatever age. Each morning I seek encouragement from my Bible. Sometimes the days and weeks are not long enough. I am blessed with excellent health and stamina.

"This is the day that the Lord hath made, let us rejoice and be glad in it." Yesterday is history, today comes only once, so each morning I rise to shine blessed with another day with whatever may be on my timetable.